GROTON PUBLIC LIBRARY
52 NEWTOWN ROAD
GROTON, CT 06340-4395

P9-DEV-510

A Bowlful
of Ladoo

Marya Ursin

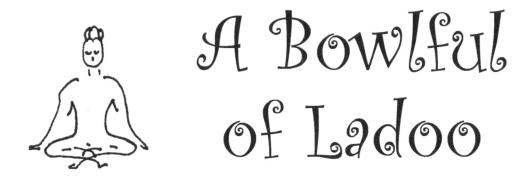

A Bowlful of Ladoo

Tales of yogic myth and form

Illustrated by Daniel Potter

with line drawings by the author

FAST BOOKS

DEC 8 – 2014
J
613.7
URS

This book is dedicated to my beloved, treasured daughter,
Ana Elliott Tiwathia, and to my amazing sister, Toasty Hancock.
May the dance go on.

Published by Fast Books, P. O. Box 1268, Silverton, Oregon 97381
ISBN 978-0-9887162-1-6
Copyright © 2013 by Marya Ursin

Introduction

I began practicing yoga at Integral Yoga on West Thirteenth Street, back when no one was doing yoga. I was a young dancer in New York City, my mind and body and spirit held together by a dream and a tribe of friends. I was on scholarship at the Merce Cunningham Studio, where I discovered time and space in ways I had never considered. It was as though my very cilia shivered at the extraordinary experience of being. I stretched, struggled, had a ceiling fall in on me, was sore, was happy.

My feet brought me to yoga: I thought I needed a world of breathing and of letting go to help me in my dancing, to help me through the various immolations that life was offering me. I had had a yoga warm-up with a visiting choreographer when I was a sophomore at Swarthmore, and it had intrigued me. When yoga came again, another world opened.

So. I have been practicing ever since—that warm-up was in 1969. We used English terms for the postures. The more exotic naming in Sanskrit was to come a couple of decades later for American yoga practice. For me, with the Sanksrit came the stories. Who was Hanuman? What warrior? Which mountain? I assumed the postures were named for natural phenomena, or for qualities. To discover the stories was an explosion into a meta experience of the yoga for me.

I live in stories. I perform in mask, and we tell stories, with the Mystic Paper Beasts. I find the stories deepen, lighten, and expand me. I began seeking stories for asana—the term for posture which means, essentially, "easy seat." My practice became brighter with these stories, which would then carry me, until it was simply the breath that was carrying me. The stories became not only a matter of laughter and curiosity, but also of liberation.

For years I have thought to make a book about a handful of these asana stories, and here, now, is the time and the place for this book, this offering. Ladoo are those very sweet dumpling confections of Indian cuisine, and they are beloved of Ganesh, the elephant god who blesses new ventures. For this reason, I call this *A Bowlful of Ladoo*—they are for you, for me, for Ganesh, for all beings.

I have more people to thank than I can name. I thank my parents and my family for birthing me into a world so extraordinary, so full of beauty and movement. I thank my most precious daughter Ana, who brought a song to my life. I thank my husband and the illustrator of this book, the ebullient Dan Potter. I thank my extended family of stepchildren, their spouses and little children. I thank my lovers of yore. I thank my cats and garden. I thank my many teachers of yoga and of dance. I thank the many articles, books, websites, storytellers, over the years, who have informed me. I thank my friends. You see, I can go on and on.

For this book, I specifically thank the following, my most generous readers, fact-checkers, and artistic counselors:

For the accuracy of the content, my friend and scholar, Dr. Serinity Young, who generously checked all my information with original sources and texts; the Hindu priestess Dr. Sunita Vaze.

For the text style, and content: Lee Kalcheim, Michael Smith.

For positive support and advice in the reading of the text: all the above, as well as Ana Tiwathia, Aditya Tiwathia, Jeff Nichols, Peter Nichols.

For paintings and sweetness, of course, my husband, Dan Potter.

For design and layout, and for offering to publish this book, Michael Smith of Fast Books Press.

I thank you all.

My life is rich and full. I offer this bowlful of ladoo to you.

Invocation to Ganesh

Ganesh! Ganesh!
Plump elephant god, remover of obstacles,
bringer of auspicious new beginnings!
I feel you present, here, and now, in this endeavor.
Bring your mischievous energy to the stories, your gaiety to the images,
your solid elephant legs to the carriage of it all.
Ganesh, I offer you ladoo, sweet dumplings, and a dance of joy!
May all beings be filled with well-being.
May all beings be happy.
May all beings be free.

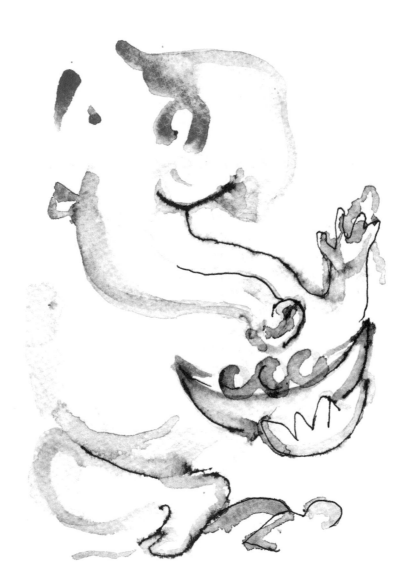

A Story about the Birth of Ganesh

Ah, Shiva, that ash-covered god! He goes off for years at a time, alone, to meditate, while Parvati, his wife, remains at home, in the green glades, creating beauty around her, awaiting the return of her husband. His silences are familiar to her, and she even misses these.

This time it has been a thousand years, and Parvati is fed up. She wants company, and family. She sits in meditation (she has known forever how to meditate), and then from the sandalwood of her skin, the dust of the earth, and the breath from her mouth, she puffs! and creates a child—Ganesha! Oh, the birds sing at the beauty of this little boy, and Parvati rejoices in his laughter and his company.

One day, when Parvati goes behind the vines to the bathing hole, she sets Ganesh at the gateway, saying, "Do not allow anyone in while I am washing my hair—I like to have my time in the bath, alone."

Ganesh stands guard as a little boy does, with fierceness—and also with eyes that see lizards and tigers and clouds, and ears that hear songs and rustles, and a nose that smells the tiger and the lamb. He is proud to be asked to do this.

But wait, who approaches in a cloud from the distance? A wild and dusty man with snakes across his chest and great matted locks of hair!

"Let me pass!" exclaims Shiva, for it is he. He feels he is at home and must not be blocked.

But Ganesh has his assignment. He exclaims, "No, sirrah, you must not pass!"

Shiva roars and demands passage again, and again Ganesh, trembling a bit now, refuses him entry.

Shiva, who is not known for his patience, takes out his sword and, in one swoop, lops off the head of the boy guarding the glade in which his mother bathes.

Off rolls the head! The little body stands, teetering.

Parvati has heard the commotion, and hastily wrapping a bright-coloured sari around herself, her dark hair wet around her face, she comes out. What is this she sees? Her darling child, headless, and her beloved husband, fuming, with his sword drawn, victory in his eyes, and a smile for his wife.

"Woe! What have you done? Slain your son!" cries out Parvati to her astonished husband. She breaks into sobs so wrenching you might think that she too would break apart.

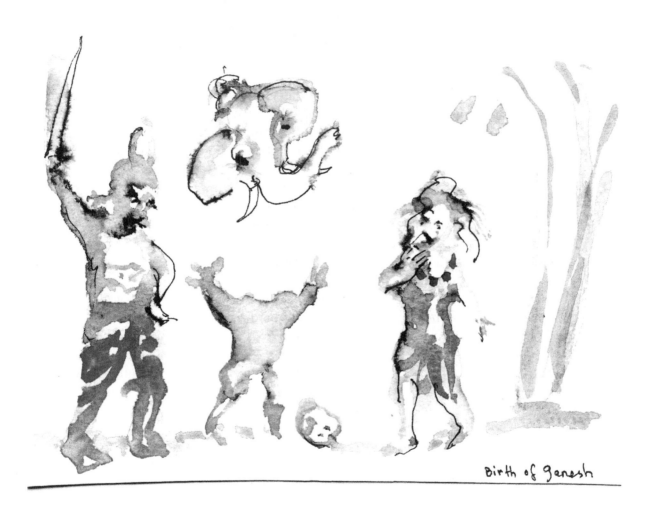

Birth of Ganesh

Shiva is appalled. "I did not know!" he protests.

Parvati looks at him with eyes full of terrible loss and says to him, "But you, you, Shiva, you are a god! Had you paused, you would have known! This is what comes of your precipitous action!!! You have destroyed our own son! So what is it you do on those long meditation trips, if you come back like this? Can you not pause and breathe for a moment before destroying what is before you?"

Shiva is stung, knowing that what she says is true. He is still impetuous. This is a good quality, too, he thinks, but not right now. What he needs to do is to find a solution. What can he do?

Another head! Ahhh, brilliant!

"The next being who comes into our vision—that head will go to our son!" declares Shiva.

An elephant appears—and boing! off comes his head—and bop! lands on the shoulders of the still-shivering little boy.

Shiva grins to see his elephant child. Parvati is stunned, but knows this to be her son, with his sweet beating heart and—his elephant head!

Not one to admit he was wrong, Shiva proclaims, "Because of this unexpected transformation, I give you, Ganesh my son, these gifts. You will be the Remover of Obstacles, the Bringer of Auspicious New Beginnings! You will be Lord of the Ganas, and you will have a mouse to ride. Your belly will be large with the generosity of life, and your ears will be able to hear all that

is good, and to separate it from that which is unkind. You are my son, Ganesha, born of your mother, Parvati, of her dreams and her joys. You will thrive and cause all others to thrive."

This was a maha blessing indeed, and it has been so ever since, that Ganesh has brought blessings to all.

Ganesh

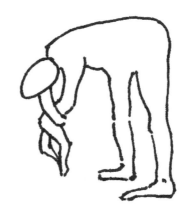

Ganesh removes obstacles from new ventures. When we wrap our arms around ourselves in a twirl like taffy, and then hang over, with the arms dangling and bound, and walk in a large, heavy-footed manner, then we evoke the steady, moving presence of the elephant-headed Ganesh. Our arms, when released, are then full of the new energy needed for new adventures.

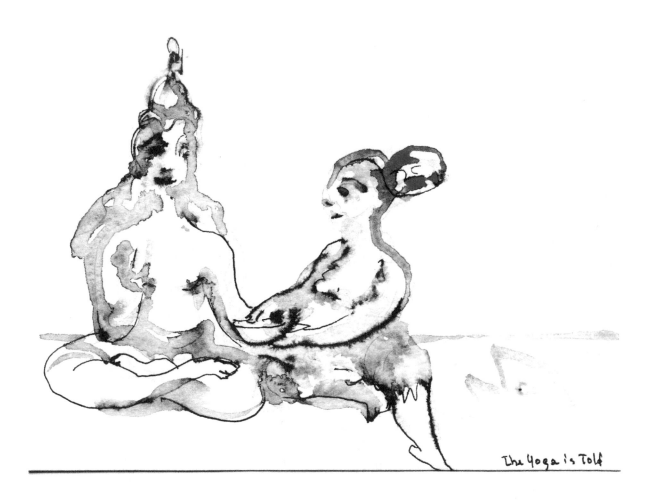

The Yoga is Told

The Yoga is Told

Once again Shiva went off, this time for ten thousand years! to meditate atop Mount Kailash. This time, he was given a great gift—the secret of freedom, the knowledge of yoga! He rushed back, hair all matted, to his beloved Parvati.

She expected him, as wives often do, and had a picnic ready.

"Oh, Shiva! Is that you, dear?" she teased, as though she did not recognize him anymore.

"Parvati! I have so much to teach you!"

"Yes, dear," she responded, giving her Shiva a kiss. "Hello, welcome home, and I love you, too."

Whoops! He always forgot about these little nice ways she has of being—like saying hello after being apart for 10,000 years! Parvati is so civilized! She is also a goddess of great wisdom, and she knows her Shiva.

Shiva paused, a bit abashed. He swept her a wide bow, saying, "Ahhh, Parvati, my love. How happy I am to see you after these many years!"

Parvati smiled. "Let us go to that little island in the sea, my love," she suggested, "and we can enjoy these delicate foods while we chat and sing together. It is so long since you have been home."

Shiva could scarcely contain himself, and he burst out, as soon as they got to the island: "Parvati! Let me tell you of yoga, of breathing and of chakras, of postures and of bliss! This is the path to freedom!" And excited Shiva discoursed on the magical gifts of yoga until the sun began to sink.

Now, Parvati had been practicing yoga for longer than she could remember, and had thought that Shiva already knew of this way to freedom. But she listened politely, a bit bemused, as she set out their picnic on that island by the river.

"Why is she not fascinated?" Shiva wondered, not knowing that all he said was like a familiar story, told again and again, to her.

A fish swimming by heard the voice of Shiva and paused. Matsya was mesmerized, and as Shiva spoke, he felt himself embodying the practice of yoga until he was one—in union!—with the practice, and with all that is. Imagine that glistening fish, wiggling and twisting and going upside down, breathing his little gills out and in. Shiva saw this, and realized that the fish was his student—his first real student! of the yoga. In exhilaration, he breathed the brahma breath and danced his Shiva dance and called on Vishnu to preserve this discovery.

Matsya, enlightened, flopped onto the island,

happy in his yoga, his gills opening to the sky, and became half a man, half a fish. Shiva called him Matsyendra, the Father of Yoga.

Parvati continues to do her yoga, and also to offer picnics and songs to Shiva, and laughs at all that is new and old, as Shiva goes off on his discoveries.

Matsyasana

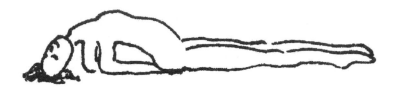

The posture of the fish, Matsya, is said to open the lungs to all that is, and to allow a yogi to float down the sacred rivers with ease, like a fish. Matsya is further special to Vishnu, who took the form of a fish to save the first human from the archetypal flood, the overwhelming life. The posture is taken on the back, with the high center of the chest lifting to the sky, as though drawn upward by a thread of desire. The head drops back, and the throat, and thyroid gland, are openly revealed.

Ardha Matsyendrasana

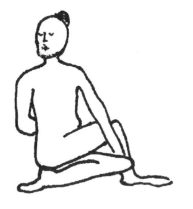

The posture dedicated to Matsyendra, the Father of Yoga, is a seated twist, so that one is taking the front part of the body to the back and the back to the front, ever illuminating conscious and unconscious, each with the light of the other. The legs are folded to represent the tail of a fish, with the upper body rising toward the sky in the twist of expanding consciousness, so one truly embodies a morphing consciousness in body form.

Warriors

Sati, graceful and beautiful, had been in love with Shiva from the time she was a tiny princess in her father's palace.

"No!" said her father, King Daksha. "Shiva is not my choice for you! Daughter—look at him! He is covered with ash, his hair is matted, and he has a reputation for going off on thousand-year meditation retreats. He can be no husband to you, my precious little daughter."

Sati was an obedient child, so she aquiesced to her father's desires—but not really. She knew she would be with Shiva. It was in her stars! she said to herself, romance in her secret sparkling eyes.

Daksha threw a party for eligible young men, and Sati met them all. They were very agreeable. When the time came for her to place a garland around the neck of the young man of choice, Sati tossed the garland up into the air and called out, "Shiva!"

Shiva plummeted down from his place in the heavens, caught the garland, and took Sati to be his wife.

King Daksha was furious, for he had no love for this fearsome god. He did not realize that his daughter, his darling Sati, was actually the goddess Shakti, and that she must be with Shiva.

Time passed. Sati and Shiva were happy, but her father stayed disgruntled.

One day Daksha gave a party, inviting one and all, everyone but Shiva. What an insult! Though incensed, Shiva determined to ignore the slight. Sati, however, wanted to go to the party, to argue her case and defend her beloved.

This did not go well. The other guests were amazed at the harsh words King Daksha had for his daughter. She pleaded with him, but to no avail.

Finally she said, "If this is how you feel, father, then I give up this physical body that you have given to me from your blood and bones."

With that, she sat down in meditation, right in the middle of the party. Her meditation was so strong that it engulfed her in flames, and she burned right up, leaving only a bit of ash behind. Her father was devastated.

Shiva, hearing of this, was full of agony and fury. He pulled at his hair and tossed a lock of it on the ground, crying, "Rise, Warrior!"

And up from the hair sprang the fiercest of warriors, whom he called Virabhadra—Vira meaning hero, Bhadra meaning auspicious. This warrior was bold and loyal, and a friend.

"Go, Virabhadra, and avenge me, and my Sati!"

In the blink of an eye, Virabhadra stood in

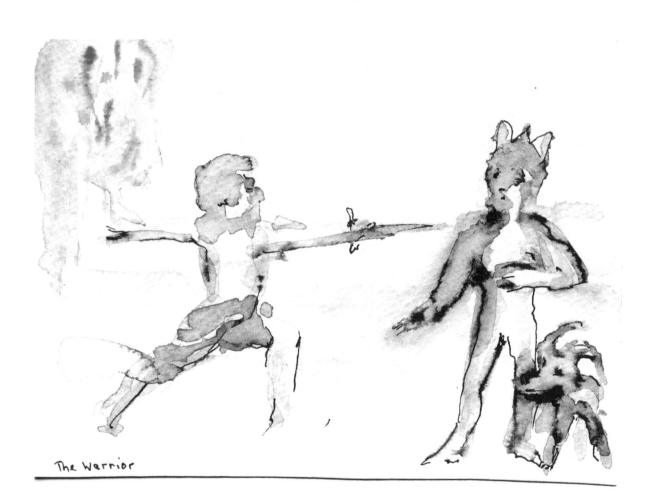

The Warrior

front of King Daksha, who was weeping for his daughter. The warrior reached out with his sword, and lopped off the king's head.

This was exactly what Shiva had wanted. But Sati, instantly reborn, rebuked him. "Shiva! Once again you have acted precipitately. Do you think that this will make Daksha like you? Do you think this will bring us peace in the family? Oh, can you not learn not to be so hasty?"

"Whoa!" thought Shiva. "She is right! What have I done?"

He zipped down to the palace of King Daksha. Aha! The story of Ganesh has prepared you for what is to come! Shiva saw the grieving and headless Daksha, and lo, out of the woods strolled—a goat! He popped the goat's head atop Daksha's body.

Somehow this made all well, and suddenly Daksha saw the worth of his son-in-law, or at least recognized the devotion of Shiva to Sati, and the three of them, Daksha, Shiva, and Sati, had a party of jubilation for new respect and friendship!

Virabhadrasana

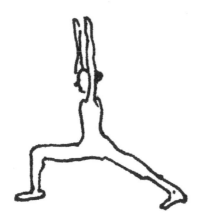

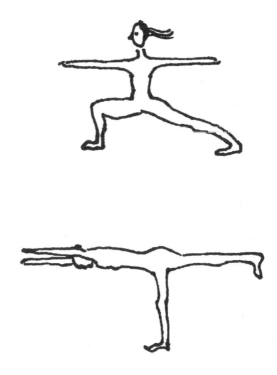

Warriors need neither lean into the past, nor leap forward into the future. They are simply present. There are three versions: one presents (Warrior I), one acts (Warrior II), and one flies (Warrior III). A firm stance allows for balance and determination.

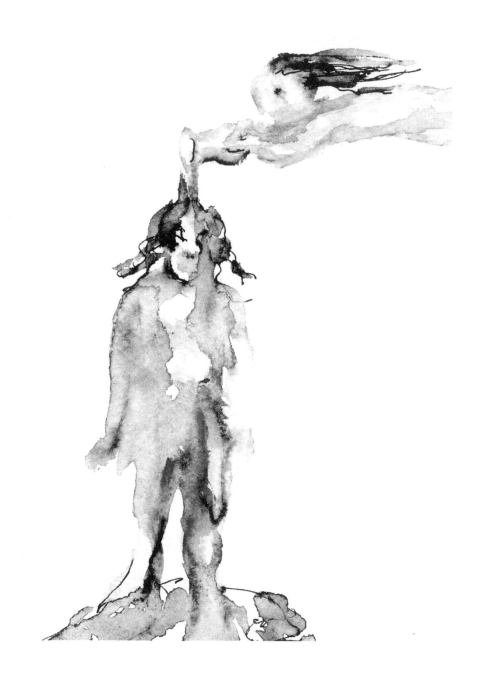

The Mountain

Shiva was not only hot-headed. He did not solve all his problems by removing heads and then replacing them with another! He could also be generous and passionate.

It used to be that the earth was all mountains, valleys, fields, oceans—there were no rivers, no waters that ran through the lands.

The Sage Bhagiratha was troubled by this. He sat and thought and thought. And—he had a brainstorm. Why not ask the heavens for more waters?

"Oh, Devi, wonderful goddess Ganga, might you come to us here, on the earth, and bring to us the wonderful flow of your waters, the rushing of your intuition, the balance of your love?"

Ganga Devi, hearing this, was flattered, and also saw the merit in Bhagiratha's request. Were she to come to earth, the earth would flourish, and this would benefit all beings. Ganga Devi turned to the gods:

"I am willing to do this! I am bold, strong, and full. I shall go to the earth and bring water, but—" and here was her condition, for many acts are easier done with help, rather than all alone! "I must have someone to break my fall from heaven. Which of you will do this?"

There was a silence amongst the gods. Then Shiva of the matted hair leapt up.

"I am Shiva! I shall, Ganga Devi, break your fall."

And down went Shiva to the earth, ready for Ganga.

There he stood, on the mountain, bracing himself, and Ganga poured her waters over his head. My goodness! such wild waters there were, and they seemed to come forever! As they hit the head of Shiva, he closed his eyes, and the waters broke into rivulets, following his matted locks of hair, streaming down, creating all the rivers of the world.

What lush green, what blessings, poured down from heaven onto Shiva's head, and onto the earth!

The Ganges River begins in the Himalayas, there on the spot on which Shiva stood. And so we have rivers and streams, running water of all kinds, here on this beautiful earth.

This time, Shiva used his own head—in a different way!

Tadasana

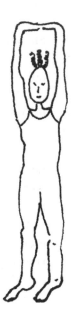

Mountain posture is grounded through the feet, and the yogi, lifting up and out through the head, reaches up to receive blessings earth to sky to earth, from soles to crown to soul!

Ganesh and the Moon

One day Shiva and Brahma were sitting together chatting. Ganesh and his big brother Kartikeya were playing around the adults. Ganesh was argumentative, claiming every toy for himself, claiming to win every contest. Then there appeared a tantalizing distraction for the little elephant-headed boy! A man came with an offering of the most delicious of fruits and sweets for Shiva. Now, you remember how much Ganesha loooooved sweets!

"Yumm! Me! Mine!" cried out Ganesh, for he was a greedy little being.

"No!" said Brahma. "Most must go to your brother, Kartikeya, as he is the elder."

Now Kartikeya did not care for sweets the way Ganesh did, but he did very much like being privileged, as the Elder Brother.

A dark cloud appeared on the brow of Ganesh. How dare his uncle Brahma tell him to share!

Oooo how Ganesh stamped his foot and fumed. Truth be told, he was already very full of sweets, but he wanted more. And—he had a point to make!

"I'll show them!" he thought. He grabbed some sweets, and said to his brother, "You will be sorry, as you may never see me again!" And he hopped on his tiny mount and sped away, as fast as a mouse can go.

Suddenly a cobra appeared!

"Eeek!"

The mouse veered sharply, and Ganesh took a spill! It was really quite comical.

Chandra, the moon, began to chortle, and then to laugh and laugh.

Ganesh looked up, furious.

"I'll show you!" (He was always showing someone!)

He broke off his tusk, ow! and flung it at the moon, which promptly went out.

"That serves the moon right," thought Ganesh, as he wrapped the cobra around his wiggly belly and trotted off home.

But soon all was sadness. With no moon, there was no night, no mystery, no romance. With no moon, the sun shone continually. With no moon, all things were parched and sad.

"What has happened? What can we do?" thought the gods.

"Squeak!" said the little mouse, and soon told all.

Agni and Indra went to Ganesh. "Please, Ganesh, forgive the moon for its laughter. Laughter is a good thing, and as I understand it, your tumble offered a bright cheerful sight! Do not take the moon away from us because of your pride!"

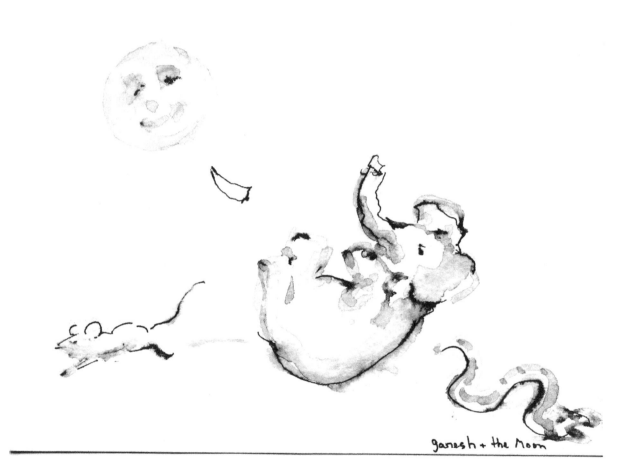

ganesh + the Moon

Ganesh, being sweet at heart, was mollified by the requests by such great gods, and said, "Yes, of course, Chandra can shine again. I love the moon, and moondrops, and moon cakes, and moonshine, and . . . but maybe the Moon could not shine on my birthday. I don't want to be laughed at like that on my birthday."

So one is not to look at the moon on the birthday of Ganesh. And a dark spot remains on the moon, where the tusk hit him and put out his light, those many years ago.

As for Ganesh, his broken tusk reminded him that he was his father's son, and given to fits of anger, in the midst of all his sweetness.

Ardha Chandrasana

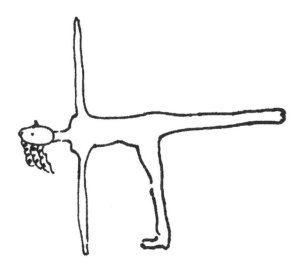

The half moon holds the glow of the full moon, balancing in her mutable way from crescent to glory. The posture is taken bravely, on one leg, tipped way over sideways, heart and back open to the full span of being, with arms reaching wide as though holding the night dream of the planets.

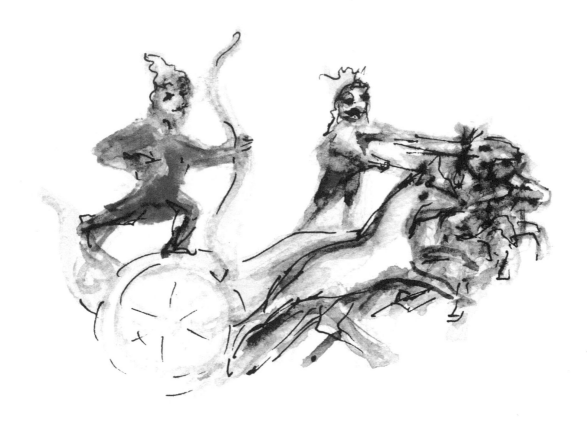

Bow

Bow: Drawn and Arched

Now that moonlight was restored, Kama, the god of love, could once again shoot his sugar-cane arrow from a bow made of honeybees, to bring that sweet sting of bliss.

But the arched bow itself is often associated with Arjuna, the greatest of archers and the hero of the Mahabarata.

"Fight!" roars the family.

"Fight!" roars the kingdom.

"Fight!" roars the inflamed mind.

There has been a great injustice, now forgotten, of course, as happens with such things. Brother fights brother, cousin fights cousin. It is not a happy time.

Arjuna is a young brother. Brave warrior that he is, he is off in a chariot, flags waving, the colors of his family bright in the morning sky. He speeds along, with full confidence that he is the greatest of archers, but in the middle of this speed, his heart hesitates.

"These are not my enemies! What am I doing? What should I be doing? If I do not do battle, my brothers, my mother, they will all be destroyed, and our honor will be as dust, but if I do fight, my cousins will die, and perhaps so shall I! What folly is this!"

He is on a chariot, his bow is drawn, the horses are galloping. His thoughts are galloping. What to do? What to do??

The warriors are ranged on either side, and the choice must be made.

It turns out that this is part of a much greater story and lesson, and it is nonc other than the god Krishna who is the charioteer! He has something to say to Arjuna, and what he says is unforgettable.

"Arjuna! You are a warrior in name, and you must be a warrior in action and thought. This is you. You do not know the larger picture, you do not know the outcome. You are a part of everything, and of nothing. It is simple: get out of the way: think not of yourself, think not of the outcome. Simply be present for all that is."

Arjuna shakes his head in confusion, and his head clears. Who is this who is speaking to him? He hears Krishna's voice and recognizes it as his own: "We come and we go. It is simply necessary to draw the bow and to let go."

And off Arjuna goes, bow drawn, with the flag of Hanuman on his chariot, leaping ever forward, not knowing what will come, brave in the present.

Shooting Bow: Akarna Dhanurasana

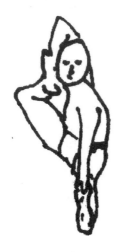 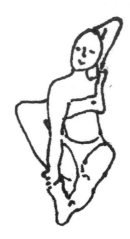

Now that moonlight is restored, Shooting Bow posture brings energy to the night. The yogi is seated, and one leg is drawn vigorously back toward the ear, while the other remains outstretched on the floor. In the second version, the foot is drawn back by the opposite hand, across the body, toward the other ear. Again, the under leg remains outstretched

Dhanurasana

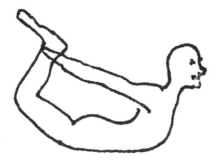

Another bow, Dhanurasana, is taken on the belly, lifting away from—and connected to—the earth, with the hands holding the ankles. We, like Arjuna, go to the furthest extreme of vulnerability and of strength, ever connected to self and to earth.

Hanuman's Red-Pepper Leap

All is lost, all is lost! So thought the monkeys and the other animals as they stood on the shore between the southernmost tip of India and the island beyond, on which—might there be? there just might be!—the beautiful Sita, the kidnapped Sita! imprisoned by the demon Rakshasa king, Ravana.

Sri Lanka was far too far away for even the most athletic of them to swim or jump, and a bridge was out of the question. Sita's husband Rama and the warriors were elsewhere battling.

Bafflement and dismay. Failure on the edge of the water. The minds of the monkeys were spinning with sadness.

Jambavantha, the wise bear, looked at Hanuman, saying, "O monkey, son of the wind, o Hanuman, remember who you are, and what you can do!"

Hanuman had been granted many boons and powers as a baby monkey—that is another story—but he was also given forgetfulness of these, so that he would not become too mischievous around the older sages. So he did not remember.

But it was true: he could change shape, he could fly, he could resist fire, and he would always be happy in his devotion.

Jambavantha gravely and a little bit desperately said again, "Remember! You must remember, Hanuman!"

"Remember, remember, remember who you are," thought Hanuman. The thought came to him like a soft chant, swirling around.

And suddenly, he leapt!

And—wow—what a leap it was! It was as though hot pepper was in his feet and jump-bouncing him across the seas, past a rising mountain, through the mouth of a sea monster, all the way to the gates of the beautiful city of Lanka, the luxurious lair of the elegant Rakshasa king.

To where there might, there just might, be the beautiful Sita.

"Remember, remember, remember!"

There in enemy territory, Hanuman shape-shifted to become a small cat, hopping onto garden walls, whisking his tail about, shivering his whiskers.

"Who is that?—a lovely young woman—could it be Sita? Pale and thin, she weeps, under the ashoka tree. It is she! Oooo how small she seems! I must not startle her," thought the kitty Hanuman. And he leapt to a branch above her.

"Sita!" he called, like the whispering leaves. "Sita! Look up!"

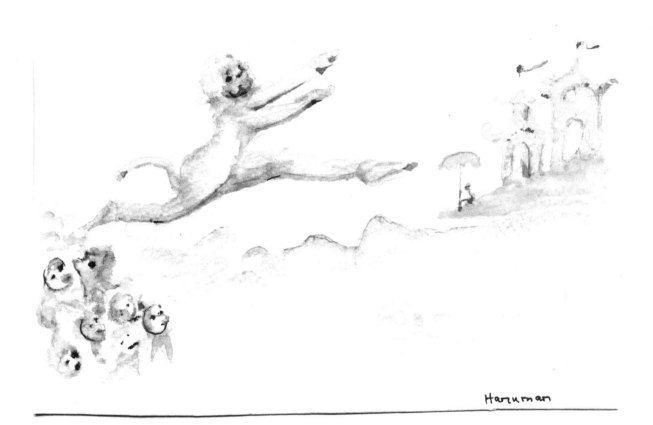

Startled, she looked up to see a small cat, a cat whose face became a monkey's face, and then again a cat. Was he a rakshasa come to torment her?

"I come from Rama, Rama, Rama! Rama will come for you, be brave, o Sita," chanted the little cat-monkey. Just to be sure, he handed Sita a ring given him by Rama, so she would be convinced.

And Sita believed him.

"Ohhhh," she breathed. "Take back this hair jewel of mine to Lord Rama, little monkey, and please, monkey, tell him to come soon, very soon, before it is too late! Go quickly, Hanuman, and be not distracted!"

Sita patted the kitty-monkey on his head, and off he went.

But Hanuman could not resist. He mocked the guards, and led them on a merry chase! He was captured by the demons, he escaped with his tail on fire, he brought down pillars and walls, and after many more mischievous exploits, naughty monkey that he was, he remembered! Sita! Save Sita! Tell Rama! Hanuman once again leapt back to the tip of India, that huge leap over waters and mountains, an impossible leap.

He took the hair jewel of Sita's to Rama. What joy! and fury! Rama's faced lighted, and then darkened. And the battle began, for Sita! to bring Sita back, once again, to her Rama.

And what of Hanuman?

"Rama Rama Rama" is written on every bone of Hanuman's little furry body, and his name is on every breath of the monkey's voiceless dreams.

Hanumanasana

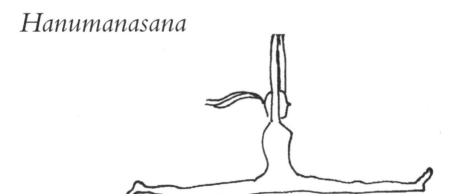

The asana that is associated with the monkey Hanuman is, as you might guess, the full split! Only so was he able to span the seas and mountains in his quest for Sita, for Rama. With this posture, the yogi reaches beyond, and leaps from one state of being to another, fearlessly, and with joy!

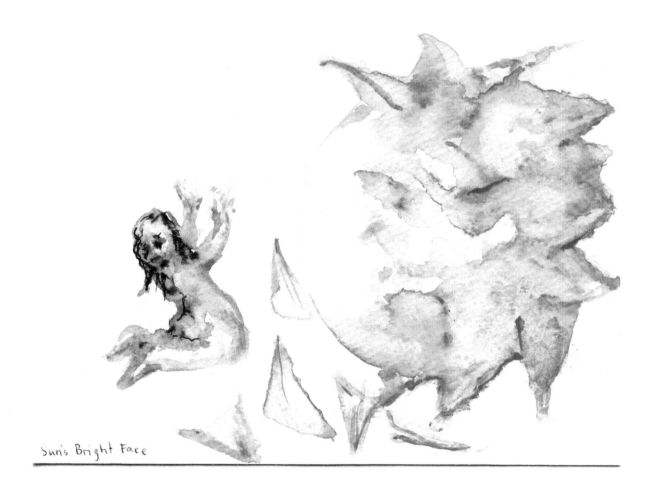

Sun's Bright Face

The Bright Fire of Love

Surya, the sun, brightly and hotly loved Sanjana. Oooo the heat was fierce!

Said she, "I love you, oh Surya, my husband, but can you shine a wee bit less brightly on my face, for I am blinded by your light!"

Sanjana was bright in her own right, but really, this was nothing compared to the brilliance and heat of the sun, for she was not a goddess of the skies, but only a human, the daughter of Vishwakarman, the gifted architect of all that is.

"My love, I am sun to all, and I do not know how to be less bright," said Surya, casting his ever-bright gaze away from Sanjana.

And the bright rays continued.

Sanjana, burned and cindered and sick at heart, ran back to her father's home, crying that she knew not what to do.

"I have left behind my shadow self, Chaya, so that Surya will not miss me, at least for a bit."

Well! Surya did not miss Sanjana! In fact, he did not even notice that this was not Sanjana, his wife, but only her shadow self. Chaya had breakfast with him, slept at night with him. In time, that sun god Surya had a son with Chaya, whom they called Shani! Uh oh.

This was not at all what Sanjana had intended. Enraged, she rushed back to her husband, called out Chaya, and made her once again a mere shadow—even less than that—a mere illusion of a shadow!

Sanjana promptly had two children with Surya. Oh yes, life was complicated for a time, with hurt feelings, confessions, banishments, and returns. There were ups and downs, bright times and shuttered ones.

"Why?" cried out the great sun, Surya.

"Ahhh," came the purring voice of Sanjana's father, the architect of all that is. "There is no fault, there is only light! My daughter, Sanjana, cannot withstand your too great brightness. That is why you now have shadows in your life."

Surya was astonished. His brightness was his gift!

"What can I do? for I am indeed the sun!"

Vishwakarman's fame as the great architect was not for nothing, and one thing that architects do is to solve problems.

"Here, let me tone down your shine a bit," said he, "and from this, we can make some spinning wheels of energy!"

And that is just what he did! He shaved off some rays from the edge of the sun. From these rays, Vishwakarman created the great many-spoked brilliant chakra wheel of the god Vishnu.

Surya regained his wife by bringing her a

face not quite so burning bright as it had been, but with a heart full of as much ardor, and all was well.

And for us, the bright sparks make spinning wheels of energy arranged in a line from earth to sky in all our bodies.

Chakrasasana

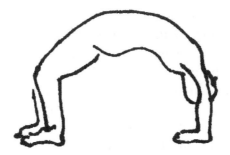

The wheel of Vishnu was said to be constructed from the many little rays that the sun released in order to be with his wife. When the yogi does the full back bend, reaching her heart to the heavens, she is taking the form of the ever bright and sparkling chakra made from the sun's fiery love.

Garuda

"What is that!? Fire!!"

"It is the end of the world!"

"It is the end of an era!"

"Fire, fire, from, oh my word, from—an Egg!"

"It is—gracious goodness me—Garuda! the son of Vinata. Good heavens, Vinata, what have you been eating!"

Garuda was born like fire from an egg, so huge and frightening that everyone thought it was the end of all time. But no, it was the bright, shining, baby eagle man.

"Garuda, my child. Everyone is fearful of your brightness. Can you make it a bit less, at least for the moment?" asked his mum, Vinata.

And so he did, for he did not want to scare others. He wanted to be good, and to take good care of his mother.

Vinata was the second wife of Kashyap, and she and Kadru, the first wife, were always in competition. One day Vinata entered a bet with Kadru and lost.

"Ha ha!" said Kadru. "You are now my slave, Vinata, and I shall leave my children to guard you!" Her children were all serpents.

Hearing of this Garuda immediately went to Patala, the abode of the snakes, where his mother was being kept. Although Garuda was fierce, he was also good at making bargains, and began a conversation with the snakes in the hopes of finding a way to free his mother. The snakes wound around one another and considered.

"O.K., Garuda, we will release your mother, foolish gambler that she is. But in return, you must bring us a cup of the elixir of immortality."

"That is impossible!" said Garuda.

"Ah, well," hissed the snakes, "if you want your mother..." and they left it at that.

No one but the gods was allowed to have this elixir. Amrita, as it was called, was kept by the gods on the top of a mountain, surrounded by leaping flames, protected by spinning blades, and guarded by two spitting serpents. Terrifying!

But Garuda, devoted to his mother, and brave down to his smallest feathers and largest bird claws, Garuda, with a swish of his wings, a diving of his body, a slashing of his beak, swooped up to the heavens. He took up the water from several rivers to douse the flames, made himself tiny to fly past the blades, and flapped his wings like crazy to blow dust in the eyes of the serpents, while he zipped in to grab the amrita in his talons.

"Amrita! I have it! My mother will be free!" But then Garuda paused in mid-flight, hovering between heaven and earth, and thought, "I cannot let those serpents have the

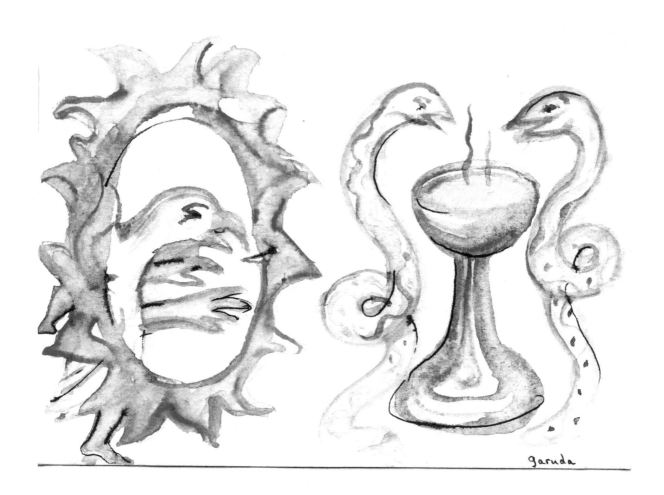

garuda

amrita! Then they, and all serpents, would be immortal! That would be terrible! What shall I do?"

Vishnu saw Garuda pause, and admired him for his thoughts that went beyond his immediate circumstances.

"Garuda," said Vishnu, "I am going to make you immortal, but the snakes, no no no! Here is what we can do." And they spoke in windy whispers, hovering there in the clouds.

Down down flew Garuda, to the nether land of the snakes, to where his mother was being kept. The snakes were thrilled to see that he carried with him a beautiful sacred vase. Amrita!

"Now we sssshalllll be immmmmorrrtallll," they hissed happily, slithering in a swarm toward the amrita.

But Garuda stopped them. "What are you thinking," he exclaimed, "to approach the sacred without having washed!"

He glared at them, and they slithered a bit less, all in a writhing clump of snakiness staring at him with malevolent, baffled eyes. "You must go cleanse yourselves before you partake of such a sacred drink. But first, first you must release my mother."

The snakes, being basically honorable creatures, agreed. Vinata emerged safe and sound. After a couple of farewell hisses and darting of tongues, the snakes dutifully went trooping off in one quick and slithering mess to bathe in the spring.

Suddenly Indra arrived and without a word swooped up the sacred nectar. The snakes slithered back lickety-split, hissing in their fury, but were only able to catch a few drops that had spilled from the vessel.

"Hissssss! Ow! Aieee!" they cried.

The drops were so powerful that they split the snakes' tongues—and snakes have had forked tongues ever since. Those few drops of amrita also granted them the appearance, and experience, of immortality by giving them the gift of changing their skins.

Garudasana

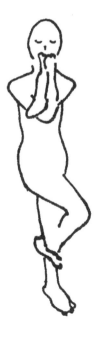

Garuda, well regarded by Vishnu, was made his sacred mount, and they say that he brings to us the vayus, the winds of breath, by which we can be liberated. The posture winds leg around leg, arm around arm, and when the yogi bends forward in this posture, the image is said to be that of the head of an eagle, with the arms being the beak, the back the bird's head, and the ears the centers of the eagle's bright eyes.

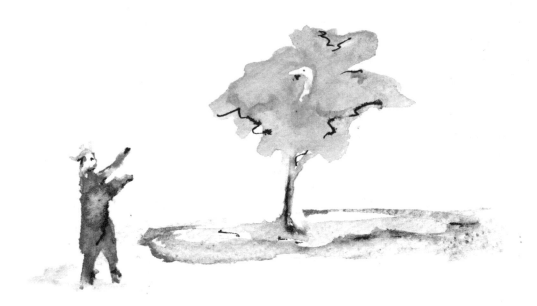

Noice in the Tree

The Voice in the Tree

W"ho is it who comes to drink from my pond?" came the voice from the tree.

The king paused, hearing the voice. He saw nothing but the lifeless bodies of his brothers, at the edge of the pond. He turned slowly around, cleverly quietly drawing his sword as he did so, and then, suddenly!! he whipped around to face—the empty pond, again.

"It must be bewitched," he thought, "or be the work of our enemies, else who could have slain five good warriors like this, at the edge of the pond?"

The voice seemed to know his thoughts, for it said, wearily, "No, young king. I am not a part of your battle, but this is my pond, and these warriors could not, nay, would not even pause long enough to try to answer my questions. Can you?" The voice sighed. Then, somberly, it continued, "If not, you too will die."

"Ask me, then, and I shall lay my heart and mind open to answer you."

The king was very thirsty. But he knew that he could slake his thirst once he had considered the questions of the voice in the tree.

What followed was amazing! Their thoughts bounced and swiveled, and laughter filled the clearing. The king forgot his thirst in the ebullience of the conversation.

"But who are you, oh wise voice in the tree?" asked the king.

"I am the Crane, here, sitting in the tree, and underneath this graceful bird's plumage, I am actually the God of Death! You, in conversing with me, have shown that you have no fear! Thank you. It is lonely being the God of Death. And this fearless regard you bring will carry you far through the forest."

The king bowed. He looked around him at his brothers' still forms, then gazed up at the Crane perched in the tree.

It was as though Crane read his thoughts: "Yes, they may again resume their lives as mortal, thirsting men. And you, dear King, you will be able to live your life fully, in the shadow of, but without the fear of, Death."

And, as the king watched, his brothers began to stir, as though just awakening, and the great Crane lifted off in that awkward lazy graceful way of cranes, flying into space. His neck stretched, his wings flapped, and he was gone

The king did not see the Crane again until one moment, many years later, when Crane appeared, bowed gravely, and lifted the king up, up, and away, a final flight.

Bakasana

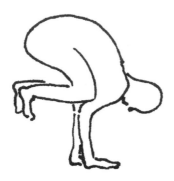

Crane perches in a tree, and the posture has the yogi stand tall and long-reaching. The arm balance posture of crow (some call it crane) requires courage and balance, and a willingness to tip forward, even if this seems dangerous to the nose!

Vishnu's couch: Ananta's pose

Vishnu lounges on his side, with one leg extended high to the sky, rather like the image of his dream of a new age coiling upwards. The yogi merges ease with stretch and dreamy expectation in this posture.

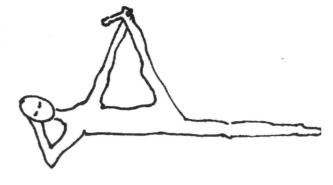

Vishnu's Dream

The act of listening begins the practice of yoga, hearing the sound that is and is not, the vast and the internal ocean of sound, of being in union—Shiva and Shakti, breathing in and out. This returns us to the dream of Vishnu at the beginning of time.

Vishnu lay on his couch of a thousand serpents, and from his navel sprouted up a blossoming lotus. In the heart of the lotus appeared the four-faced Brahma, the god of creation. Brahma sang from each of his four mouths "ah-oo-mm" and "   " (silence).

All being shivers with song, and snakes—without ears—attend these vibrations. The yogi trains to hear more deeply, to hear beyond what is known, to remembering our true nature.

Cobra rears up to hear and to remember.

Shiva, in his dance, wears the cobra. He embraces fearless transformation—from dark to light, from prison to freedom. He dances his dance to his drum of time, within a halo of flame. The flame goes on, round and round, samsara, birth and life and death and birth again, disintegrating with each beat of the drum, each new beginning. Shiva the cosmic dancer spins us to possibility, to Vishnu dreaming at the beginning of time, the lotus, the faces of Brahma, the om, the silence.

All things begin, and end.

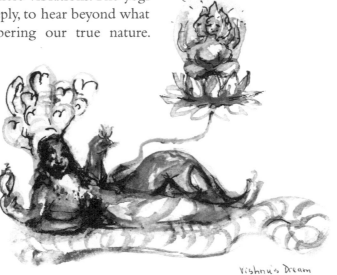

Vishnu's Dream

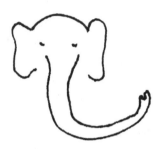

May all beings be at peace, may all beings be filled with well-being, may all beings be free.

CPSIA information can be obtained at www.ICGtesting.com
Printed in the USA
BVOW10s0612041213

338086BV00002B/2/P

9 780988 716216